DETOX
with
EASE

Detox Your Body,

Purify Your Life

Feel Great, Look Great, & Be Great!

Written by Eve Hennessa

Edited by Sarah Joy Albrecht

www.DetoxTheBodyMCS.com

Copyright © 2016 Eve Hennessa

All rights reserved.

ISBN-13: 978-1523815647
ISBN-10: 1523815647

Dedicated to the pristine beauty of the Earth and the health of all living creatures.

Thanks to all of those with chemical sensitivity, sick building syndrome and environmental and toxic illness who know directly the effects of everyday chemicals.

Joe Izzo whose kindness and expertise with brain retraining and releasing emotional toxins were essential.

Eliza who was this book's biggest encourager.

Patricia Kirk who has shared her vast knowledge of nutrition, sauna, fitness, and health.

To my mother and father who supported my entrepreneurial endeavors.

Bennie LeBeau, Bavado who encouraged this book, taught me energy clearing, and more.

Harry Lopez who was always there when every possible chemical in any situation had me coughing, irritable, and running for the nearest exit.

Bella Rosenberg, my first acupuncturist, whose skill and kindness came at just the right moment.

To Ed and Barbara P., loyal guardians of the dreamers.

Detox With Ease-
CONTENTS

1	Introduction	7
2	Toxicity and the Detox Organs	15
3	Eating and Drinking	24
4	Different Kinds of Toxins	31
5	Neurotoxins	34
6	Cleaning Chemicals	38
7	Home and Household Materials	41
8	Clothing	44
9	Personal Care Products	46
10	Dentistry	47
11	Endocrine Disruptors & Your Hormones	48
12	Electromagnetic Frequencies (EMFs)	50
13	Bacteria, Yeasts, Candida and Parasites	53
14	Stress, Emotions and the Energy Field	55
15	Detox Therapies and Considerations	61
16	Detox Side Effects: "Herxheimer Effect"	72
17	The Quick Fix	74
18	Happiness & Well Being	76
	CONCLUSION	77

Eve Hennessa

This is a Fast read and reference guide.

Most comprehensive detox info available for long term detoxification.

Contains effortless to advanced techniques.

Reduce toxins by 90% by making simple changes

1 INTRODUCTION

With a little knowledge and changing a few habits, cut your toxicity in half!

Eliminating toxins is a crucial factor in recovering from serious illness, brain function, avoiding serious illness and feeling great. You can learn how to clean out most toxic chemicals from your body without much effort. Once you know where and how to avoid toxins, detoxing is not so much work. This is the most effective and easiest detox method! And the only one that truly works.

Why learn about toxins?

Toxins are weakening the immune systems of many and causing cancer, obesity, and mood disorders in millions of people and animals.

No cleanse or method on the market is going to reduce toxins in your body effectively for long. We are taking in new toxins on an hourly basis. The key to detox is to not take in new toxins!

Toxins come into our bodies though the digestive system, through eating and drinking. We take toxins directly into our blood stream through the lungs and the skin. Emotions, situations, and attitudes also greatly contribute directly to the level of toxicity on our bodies and beings.

Detoxing requires a working knowledge of the many ways we take in new toxins, as well as how to rid ourselves of existing toxins. We will never be toxin free, but we can have our organs and systems running very efficiently so that the toxins we do have will do minimal harm.

Toxicity is an underlying factor or cause in cancer, multiple sclerosis, diabetes, fatigue, depression, heart disease, fibromyalgia, viral load, obesity, aches, asthma, pains, auto-immune illness, multiple chemical sensitivity, infertility, erectile dysfunction, anxiety, and every possible illness.

Almost every element of modern life is full of harmful toxins. With education, we can get control of the toxins we take in. There is little regulation of the chemicals found in non-food items. It's a jungle out there!

Moreover, the chemical levels found in food have rarely been studied for safety for more than a month or two. Those chemicals which have been found to cause cancer and illness are somehow deemed acceptable. They study the effect of one little chemical. There have not been studies on the effect of the hundreds of chemicals we take in on a daily basis. So far, combined toxins have been shown to have multiplied ill effects on health. It's like mixing drugs.

There is a lot of info in this short book. It takes plenty of time and many changes in order to detox to the maximum level. Keep a copy of this book on hand and study it often. Do what you can to change your lifestyle, at a pace that is comfortable to you. The real detox is not a quick fix, but a lifestyle change combined with the basic knowledge of detoxification techniques.

About Me and Chemical Sensitivity

A few years back I was a healthy person, eating organic foods and exercising daily, when I suddenly developed multiple chemical sensitivity (MCS). The scent of people's laundry detergents and perfumes felt suffocating and irritating from across the room. Within a few months I became so ill that I could not be around any air-born chemicals, which meant I could not leave the house. I developed fatigue, rashes, neurological symptoms of brain fog, reduced brain function, irritability, anxiety, twitches, numbness, and memory loss. I also developed asthma, chronic cough, and chronic lung pain. I had aches and pains and other odd symptoms. I felt old and tired. My body was breaking down at an alarming rate.

Any neurotoxic scents like laundry detergent, cleaning products, candles, air fresheners, and car exhaust would make me immediately very ill. My body was no longer able to tolerate the smallest amount of these toxins.

This MCS is a life threatening and nightmarish illness, where even the lightest amount of perfume on someone will be experienced like being sprayed you in the face with Raid. My MCS was a moderate case. Many people with this condition must go live outside miles away from car exhaust. The toxic environment causes intestinal problems, weakened organs, nervous system problems, and weakened immune system.

Politics, and brainwashing by the chemical manufacturers, have created a state where there is almost no public information on damaging chemicals in everything from Teflon to baby clothes, and anyone who brings up the subject can be seen as hippy fringe. Friends, family, and doctors alike labeled me as neurotic.

The idea that "chemicals are helpful and don't hurt you" is still accepted by most people. Anyone who has a problem with chemicals is thought to have it because of an "allergy" or is a hypochondriac. That puts the fault onto the one being affected. Chemical allergy is not really an allergy, but the body being damaged by the chemicals. It is a reaction to toxins. It is your intelligent body's alarm warning system.

In order to get well, I needed to know the toxicity of everything I came into contact with. For years, I studied the toxicity of everything. I spent countless hours researching and making phone calls to companies that produce every conceivable product from cheese to backpacks.

Years were spent studying and trying various daily healing techniques. I studied every organ and body system, including emotional and energy fields. I passed countless healing hours in the forest and became a nature mystic and studied and practiced many forms of spiritual healing.

I could not find one person that had ever healed from MCS. It is a deadly, life stopping illness and I was not going to accept that. I was determined to get well.

When my body was finally functioning much better, I had to retrain my brain to not go into the anxiety (fight or flight) response at every little synthetic smell. I was so afraid of chemicals that it took a while to be able to not sweat and panic at every smell.

After I learned everything about toxins, I needed to make peace with them and not dwell on the injustice and insanity of this state of affairs. Even though I am aware of the toxic chemicals in

everything, I am not alarmed or upset by it anymore. I believe that once humanity is informed, we will not use the toxic chemicals anymore in such large numbers. There is no need for toxins. We can keep some toxic chemicals to make life easier and better and get rid of the majority, which really aren't helping us at all.

Now I avoid toxic chemicals when possible and keep my body as pure as is comfortable for me. Everyone is going to have a different level of comfortability with toxins.

This chemical sensitivity gave me, and all others with MCS, a super-human ability to detect toxins. I could smell toxins in someone's deodorant from five feet away. It was very unpleasant, but useful information in the long run. This hypersensitivity empowers us to know what is toxic. They call those with MCS canaries in the coalmine. I never call anyone that, but it is a good metaphor.

Pretty much everything manufactured or grown in "conventional" ways is toxic. *The good news* is the human body is equipped to neutralize and excrete toxins.

If you are well, you have the leisure of picking and choosing what toxins are easy for you to give up. When your metabolism and organs are functioning well, cutting back on toxins will greatly increase your health and vitality.

If you are ill, detoxing is a full time job!

The Goal in Detoxing

The goal of detoxing is to "LIGHTEN THE TOXIC LOAD" of the body. The "Toxic Load" is the total accumulated toxins in your body.

If your body is clogged with toxins, your liver and other detox organs will not be able to process new toxins that you are exposed to. The lighter your toxic load, the better all of the organs will function and the easier it will be to feel good, strong, beautiful, and healthy.

In the process of detoxing and healing you will learn how to better listen to what your body wants. Listen to it. **If there is any food, herb, or supplement which you have doubts about using, it is best to leave that out until you have investigated it further**. Every body is different and some people are more sensitive than others.

The Detox Process is 3-fold:

1) Take in as few toxins as possible on a permanent basis.

2) Eliminate the toxins that are already in the body.

3) Enhance the health of all of your systems so that your body is functioning at an optimal level and can easily process toxins.

Eve Hennessa

Disclaimer:

None of this is medical advice. I have no medical degree whatsoever. This is information I learned along the way in my own self-healing. We are all different. Healing is a very individual process, not everything is good for everybody. Use your own discretion.

Claimer:

There is nothing here that I have not deeply investigated or used myself.

I have invested countless hours reading up on all of the disclaimers and warnings about all therapies and products mentioned herein. I firmly believe everything here to be gentle and effective. You can read a scary story about almost any subject on the internet.

Sensational negative stories get more views and should be considered accordingly. Always investigate for yourself.

Modern doctors have little or no training in everyday chemicals, nor training about nutrition and wellness in general. There is a lot of pressure on them to stick to a certain knowledge base. Doctors have other knowledge that I am very thankful for. In the long term care of our bodies, we will benefit by educating ourselves.

2 TOXICITY AND THE DETOX ORGANS

What is Toxicity?

Toxicity is literally how poisonous a substance is. Some things are very poisonous, and even a small amount can be dangerous. Many substances are only slightly poisonous, so that small amounts can be consumed without harm.

If you have an accumulated exposure to these milder poisons, like pesticides or synthetic fragrance, over time they can overwhelm your ability to detoxify (rid your body of these substances). This creates a toxic state.

Furthermore, an exposure to several mild toxins at once is much more dangerous than one at a time. It's like mixing pharmaceuticals; thus creating a toxic soup.

This is the environment we live in every day. The alarming rate of cancer, obesity, depression, and other chronic illness, is a result of daily exposure to toxins that are considered safe.

Our body is our friend and when toxic chemicals come in, our fat cells take on the job of storing these harmful chemicals in fat tissues in order to protect our vital organs. This is one of the factors why obesity is a prime factor in illness and why so many people are struggling with this condition. It is a form of toxicity. Both obesity and toxicity are linked to metabolism.

Bones and other tissues also store toxins. Over time, poisons are stored in our tissues, becoming an ongoing source of poor health.

The body must constantly work overtime to process the chemicals and starts to break down. When the organs are clogged with toxins, chronic conditions and illness arise.

Toxins come in two broad categories: *external* toxins, which are environmental, and *endogenous* toxins, which your own body makes. Environmental toxins include things like heavy metals, pesticides, chemicals, drugs, and bacterial and microbial toxins. These are present in the air, water, and food that we consume.

Toxins made by your own body include hormones, stress chemicals, and those produced by bacteria in your digestive system. Chronic stress produces some of the most damaging of toxins in the body.

A Few Symptoms of Toxicity

Toxins get stored in the brain causing depression, brain fog, and more. Toxins accumulate in the joints and at injury sites, causing aches and pains. Fibromyalgia is one of the new epidemic illnesses characterized by chronic pain and is associated with toxicity in the muscles and nerves.

Any disease can be made worse by toxicity; however, some of the most common signs and symptoms of too much toxicity in the body include:

•Recurrent headaches

•Brain fog

• Muscle aching and weakness

• Joint pain

• Nerve pain or numbness

• Recurrent infections

• Poor short-term memory and concentration

• Candida

• Sensitivity to environmental chemicals, odors, and/or foods

• Chronic fatigue and lethargy

• Anxiety, depression, mood swings

• Rashes

• Cancer

• Breathing problems

• Infertility, hormonal imbalance, erectile dysfunction

Many chronic illnesses and conditions are associated with excess toxins in the body: Chronic Fatigue Syndrome, cancer, lupus, multiple sclerosis, arthritis, infertility, erectile dysfunction, obesity, Multiple Chemical Sensitivity, and more.

Know Your Detox Organs and Digestive System

The Liver

The liver filters toxins out of the bloodstream and processes them so that they can be excreted via your bowels or urine. Optimal liver function is important for efficiently removing toxins from your body.

Milk thistle, dandelion, glutathione and coffee enema are great for cleaning the liver. Also, reduction of incoming toxins will help your liver to stay healthy and able to detox. Avoid pesticides, hydrogenated oils, and other heavy toxins to free up your liver.

The Kidneys

Kidneys are a vital detox organ. The toxins that are processed by the liver are excreted via the kidneys into the urine. More substances are eliminated from the body via the kidneys than by any other route.

Having clean water is important for kidney health. Spend time and investigate how to get the best water you can. It is well worth it. I was using a reverse osmosis water filter, but now drive to a natural spring once a month to bring water home. Distilled water is also beneficial.

Anything that comes in a plastic bottle has toxins. This is especially true if it is new plastic or plastic that has been subject to warm temperatures in the delivery truck or processing site.

Plastics are unregulated and can have just about anything in them. BPA and phthalates are just scratching the surface of the chemicals in plastics. Finding clean water can be a difficult task, but with some thought and research, you can find the best water for your lifestyle and budget. The body is mostly made up of water and it helps to have the best quality we can afford.

Recently I have read a great deal about distilled water and feel it is a good choice. Cook with pure water if possible.

Talking kindly to your water has proven to positively affect the molecular structure. So, if you can't afford the good filters for now, that is a great option.

Some people put their water in the sun in a glass container. Sun eliminates many toxins and bacteria, as well as charging it with its powerful energy. They call it "sun-charge water".

The Lungs

The lungs are an important detoxification organ. Every time you exhale, you are excreting toxins. Make sure to have the best air quality in your living environment by using plants and/or air purifiers.

Breathing exercises are incredibly detoxing. Just becoming aware of your breathing and making it as deep and slow as possible is very detoxifying and the oxygen you bring in is also great for your health. Every time you exhale, you are releasing toxins.

Time spent in nature, breathing in oxygen is a great detox. Walking out of doors is helpful. Even in cities, indoor air pollution is usually much worse than the air outside, with the exceptions of wafting laundry chemicals and diesel engines. There are many ways to detox the lungs found on my website (detoxthebodymcs.com).

Yoga, dance and other exercises opening the ribcage are great, as well as all heavy or deep breathing.

The Skin

The skin is the body's largest detox organ. The epidemic of rashes and skin conditions is not an 'allergy', but your body eliminating toxins. This is why creams don't fix chronic skin conditions.

Toxins enter the blood stream directly through the skin. They are not filtered by the liver nor broken down by digestive enzymes, like occurs when you eat something. This is why skin patch medications are so effective. The medication goes right into your blood via the skin.

Clothing, especially when new, is full of toxins. Wear organic clothes when possible. Clothing is usually sprayed with pesticides before coming from China and also sprayed with formaldehyde for preventing wrinkles and mold. Fungicides and other chemicals are also used. The chemicals in dyes and materials are what give clothing that new smell. Sadly, cotton is usually GMO and full of Roundup pesticide.

Wash all new clothes a few times before wearing. Wash clothes in baking soda or some other natural detergent. Avoid toxic lotions, shampoos, and soaps with ingredients you can't pronounce. Start to educate yourself about the toxins in clothing, products, and cosmetics. This will go a long way in helping you to detox your body. Make-up can be a source of lead and other highly toxic substances that enter in through the skin.

It is easy to make your own moisturizers with natural oils, like coconut, that actually nourish your body.

The Digestive System

Most people with toxicity issues have a condition called "leaky-gut syndrome", which is increased intestinal permeability, or small leaks in your digestive tract. In a healthy digestive system, the lining of the digestive system is a very good filter, allowing

 beneficial nutrients like vitamins and amino acids to pass into the bloodstream, while keeping toxic bacteria and the waste products of digestion within the intestines to be excreted (pooped out).

This lining in the digestive system is easily damaged by infection, toxins, and medications. Especially damaging are antibiotics, anti-inflammatory medications, and pain killers. The digestive system is also damaged by stress, "bad" bacteria, yeasts, parasites, and GMOs.

When the gut gets leaky, what happens is that partially digested foods and waste make it into the blood stream. This puts a tremendous stress on the other detoxification organs.

Eventually, some of this toxic material slips past the liver and kidneys and ends up entering the general circulation, where it can lead to many of the symptoms of toxicity. "Leaky gut syndrome" results in a great deal of stress upon the immune system, the liver, and virtually every other organ.

It is possible to have a leaky gut and not be aware of any "digestive" problems. Besides leaking toxins, leaky gut makes it difficult to get nutrition from your food. It's a very common condition contributing to poor health.

I was malnourished and did not really have any symptoms until I became ill. Even though I ate organic and very well, I was not absorbing the nutrition from my food. Swollen abdomen, pains, and common digestive issues are the usual symptoms. I did not have much of that because my diet was so good, but I did have malnutrition symptoms.

Eve Hennessa

3 EATING AND DRINKING

What You Eat

I avoid the use of the word 'diet'. It brings up so many ideas of restrictions, shame and failure. I think most diets are useless and not enjoyable at all. Food is one of life's most wonderful pleasures, and scared as such. Pleasure is a healing force, so eating healthy food that you enjoy is really an incredible detox.

That said, what we eat is very important and it is really wise to eliminate toxins and unhealthy foods as much as possible. Improving the quality of the food we eat will provide more taste and satisfaction from eating.

Eating well involves buying or growing high quality food and spending a little time in food preparation. The more pre-made and pre-packaged your food is, the more likely the quality is to go down.

Everyone is at a different level of food knowledge. Please don't be overwhelmed by the changes you may want to eventually make. Every small change is a step in the right direction. Try to enjoy this process. If you don't, you may not get too far. Remember, *Detox with Ease!*

Find new foods that you enjoy, and cook them in the way that you enjoy. Don't believe all of the diet hype out there. Focus on quality and enjoyment and spend money on the good stuff! You don't have to fast or become raw or vegan to be healthy. Those practices are good for some people, but let your body tell you what to eat.

I like southern style collard greens cooked with bacon fat and other comfort foods from my childhood. Before I realized that that is a very nutritious food, I would buy kale and it would always rot in the fridge, because I did not like it. At that time, I thought I had to eat everything raw to get the enzymes. It is great to eat raw foods, but they are actually hard to digest. I prefer quasi-paleo style eating. I eat lots of healthy fats and lots of vegetables, not so much carbs and not too many sweets. I love fruit and occasional potato chips! I always cook organic and grass-fed and love food so very much. No one will ever convince me fruit or natural cheese is bad!

Make small improvements and discover new foods that you like!

I think pleasure is the key to the French being famous for their slim figures and health, while they eat the most 'fattening' and 'unhealthy' foods on the list. I believe it is because they use the best quality and freshest ingredients, and they passionately enjoy eating.

Here are some basics to reduce or eliminate:

>Artificial colors, flavors, additives, stabilizers, and flavor enhancers, as well as foods containing hydrogenated fats, or any type of vegetable oil except olive. This information is usually contained in the ingredients list on the food label.

>Reduce sugars. Sugar can be in the form of glucose, sucrose, fructose, corn syrup, maltodextrin, dextrose, malt syrup,

molasses, maltose, lactose, and more. Corn sugars are the most unhealthy of the sugars. Replace sugar with raw honey, raisins, and fruit, and then try not to over-eat them.

Use healthy oils: coconut, and organic or known origin olive oil. If not certified organic, canola oil, soy oil, and corn oil are

> GMO, full of pesticides, and very unhealthy. Of course hydrogenated oils are better completely eliminated. Cooking with healthy oils can dramatically improve your health.

Lots of restaurants and all chains use these cheap oils. That is why it is good to prepare your own food.

> Avoid GMO food, which includes all corn and soy that is not organic.

> GMO food has shown to be responsible for many digestive and other issues which are causing a decline in general health. There are more and more GMO foods being approved. Periodically, check to see what the latest GMO foods are. GMOs cause cancer and hurt the digestive system. Also GMOs usually have a heavy load of pesticides.

More considerations:

Fresh vegetable juice makes a great addition to the detox diet.

If you own a juicer, try juicing carrots, apples, ginger, fresh beets, celery, and lemons.

Explore super foods and get plenty of organic vegetables.

Eat organic and grass-fed meat and dairy products. Grass-fed animals have nutrients not found in factory farm meats, cheese, butter, and eggs. The sun, the grass, and the air give animals a very complex and healthy nutrient composition. Grass-fed butter is a super food with Vitamin K and other nutrients. 'Organic' butter from factory cows is not a super food.

Lack of sun, overcrowding, and dirty and traumatic conditions make for toxic animal products. Wild meats are the healthiest.

Most lamb is from Iceland or New Zealand, not fed hormones, antibiotics, or GMOs, and is grass-fed. This is an excellent meat choice.

Get to know a farmer at a farmers market and get the best meats and dairy that you can. They say you are what you eat and I try not to ever eat sad, confined animals; but rather, animals lovingly and respectfully farmed.

I buy "pasture-raised" organic eggs. That way the chickens are not eating GMO corn feed. "Cage free" is not good enough.

Avoid chain restaurants: All franchise restaurants use mass-produced ingredients and serve poor quality food.

Eve Hennessa

One day I *googled* the ingredients for a Subway sandwich—I have not been tempted to eat since. They even had corn syrup and hydrogenated oils in the meat and bread. They also had other toxic ingredients in that healthy looking sandwich.

> Add lots of herbs and herbal teas and green teas to your diet. Most herbs help the body detoxify. They help tone the organs.

Rosemary, dandelion, and milk thistle are famous detox herbs. Ginger, garlic, goldenseal, and turmeric are famous for cleansing the body.

If you research enough you will find that almost any food is unhealthy—even beans, rice, or raw or cooked veggies. I say, *eat what you think your body wants*.

Above all: Enjoy your Food!

Try new things little by little. Our tastes do change as we detox addictive chemical laden foods. As we come into balance, we will crave the food that is the most medicinal for us.

• Many processed foods are purposely made with addictive ingredients, so you eat the whole box and go back for more. It may take some time to wean off of them. Go easy on yourself while changing the diet.

• Fruits are rich in essential enzymes and nutrients for detoxification support.

- Vegetables are a crucial component of any detoxification program. They are alkalizing and a wonderful source of fiber, antioxidants, vitamins, minerals, and phytonutrients, all of which support detoxification on many levels.

- Try to cut back on grains. Many people find that eliminating wheat from the diet improves their well-being. I quit eating wheat for a month experiment and now my stomach often cramps up or swells when I do eat it.

If you would like more help, I do wellness and weight loss coaching. Email *evespotofgold@gmail.com*. I can help you make realistic changes to your eating practices. You will enjoy your food, lose weight and feel great!

No counting calories, sugars, or anything unpleasant. One of the joys of adulthood is that we don't have to eat our peas if we don't want to. We are free to eat what we like.

There is always a way to find a healthy food that we like.

Water

Tap water contains many toxic chemicals such as:

- Industrial fluoride (as opposed to the naturally occurring mineral)

- Residues from pharmaceutical drugs not filtered by the water treatment system

Eve Hennessa

- Chlorine

- PVC and lead from pipes

- Water treatment processing chemicals

There are a lot of advertisements for water filters. I think that Reverse Osmosis water is the best of the filtered water, followed by distilled. I get my water from a natural spring, and bring it home in mostly glass containers. That is the best water for me. Make sure your spring gets tested now and then. Don't use the spring right after a heavy rain.

Mineral water in glass is also very good. Pellegrino has the best mineral content of top selling commercial waters. Many swear by distilled water and I think they have a point. Also alkaline water is very good.

4 DIFFERENT KINDS OF TOXINS

Plastics and Packaging

Food and drinks sold in plastic bottles contain plastic residue. This is toxic.

BPA and phthalates are only two known causes of cancer and hormone disruption. The rest of the plastic chemicals have not even been studied. Even veggie plastic is full of pesticides and GMO corn. GMO food uses very dangerous amounts of Monsanto's *Roundup*. This pesticide is wreaking havoc on health and Earth and is to be avoided always.

I probably went a year without ever drinking from a plastic bottle. It just required planning, creativity, and looking a little "different" now and then. I still rarely buy any plastic bottled drinks for environmental and health reasons.

I take my own champagne glass to art openings or parties that I go to. Everyone else is drinking from plastic and wants to know where I got my beautiful glass. I got it from my purse, of course. Be a trend setter and bring your own glass! Alcohol is a solvent, so it will leach a lot of toxins from your plastic cup.

Traditional plastics are petroleum based.

Studies show that all food inside of plastic packaging contains chemical residues from plastics. The plastic chemicals contaminate foods that were not even touching the packaging.

Spend the extra money to buy food in glass jars and to buy veggies that are not in plastic packaging. It is impossible to eliminate plastics, but you can cut back by at least 75% with a little awareness.

Seriously making an effort to avoid plastic packaging will do a lot to lighten your total toxic load.

We get a lot of unregulated materials from China that contain every conceivable poison. It's a toxin free for all out there! Limit the buying of things when you don't know what it is made of.

Cookware

One of the easiest ways to cut down on toxins is to change your cookware. One of the most toxic substances on Earth is Teflon. The FDA tried to ban it, but the industry is so profitable that it was not possible. The PFOA chemicals in Teflon can stay in the body and the environment for 20 years or longer. Heating this toxic substance causes the release of these chemicals in to the air and your food. It can even kill pet birds.

When I suffered from chemical sensitivity, I could not be in the same house with Teflon cooking without getting sick. It's a very strong poison.

Teflon is also in lots of camping gear, clothing, food packaging, etc. Toxic PFOAs are also found in the linings of microwave popcorn bags, pizza boxes, and potato chip bags. The PFOAs are what make the inside of the box or bag smooth and shiny. Popcorn is the most toxic because of the time it spends in the microwave at high heat. PFOAs cause cancer and hormonal imbalance.

Use stainless steel, glass, wrought iron, and ceramic. Even these need investigation before purchase if possible. It is almost all from China and not regulated. There is actually an "acceptable" level of radioactive waste that can be used in eating utensils. I use old sterling silver for eating. It is best not to heat up any kind of chemicals, like cheap or plastic spoons. Heating releases the toxins.

Aluminum is also very toxic. For cooking, stick to stainless steel, ceramic, and wrought iron.

As for food packaging, styrofoam is very toxic, especially drinking hot beverages from it. Plastic wrap has BPA and is not good for food storage. Aluminum foil has aluminum and other toxins. One reason I started cooking my own food was to avoid the packaging.

Eve Hennessa

5 NEUROTOXINS

A neurotoxin is a substance that is toxic to the neurons, nervous system and/or brain. They are one of the most under-emphasized poisons plaguing humanity today.

They are usually in the form of scented products and other toxins that have a smell or scent. These toxins come in to your blood stream through the nose.

To anyone who has had chemical sensitivity or chemically induced asthma, encountering everyday neurotoxins in the air in almost every building and household is a nightmare. The neurotoxic smell of Febreze makes some people go into convulsions! People have died from scented air fresheners. These days many people are becoming unable to tolerate these chemicals.

The problem with neurotoxins is that you have no choice but to breathe these in when they are present. It is not like food, which you may decline to eat.

People have almost no knowledge of the serious health problems that neurotoxins pose. Most buildings are sealed up without proper ventilation and more and more products flood the market to give you that "fresh" scent.

People are constantly bombarded with commercials and shamed into thinking that everything is cleaner if it has a chemical fragrance. Really, the true 'fresh clean scent' is no scent at all!

Take out your trash regularly, instead of buying scented trash bags. Most people clean now by adding a lot of "clean smelling" products to their dirty homes and clothes to cover the mold and other smells.

Smells are there to indicate something needs taking care of, not to be covered up.

Neurotoxins go in through the nose, right into the blood stream and the brain. This affects the brain and the nervous system. Anxiety, depression, fatigue, irritability, brain fog, Multiple Chemical Sensitivity, and erectile dysfunction are a few common conditions caused by neurotoxins.

Illnesses of the nervous system are now epidemic. We are breathing in neurotoxins through laundry detergent, perfumes, shampoos, air fresheners, automobile and diesel exhaust, house paints, chlorine in water, and common cleaning products.

Not all neurotoxins are inhaled through the nose, including: mercury, led, fluoride, mold, Botox, MSG. and Aspartame.

Most people have no idea that their poor mood may be caused by neurotoxins. Eliminate neurotoxins from your life and watch your energy level, focus, mood, and brain function improve. Many types of nervous system disorders can be caused by neurotoxicity, including numerous neurologic and psychiatric disorders.

If it is synthetic and it has a scent or odor of any kind, it is neurotoxic and/or carcinogenic. While breathing in chemicals now and then probably won't hurt you, be aware of the toxins you are breathing in and take measures to minimize them.

Open windows, keep your things clean and aired-out so they don't need covering up by sprays and fresheners.

Especially avoid synthetic scented shampoos, perfumes and laundry products. These are on your body and hair and you breathe them in 24 hours a day. Most commercial products are carcinogenic, neurotoxic, hormone disrupting, etc.

Some common neurotoxins are: adhesives, ammonia, Botox, arsenic, benzene, carbon monoxide, carpet cleaning agents, chemical warfare agents (contributing to "Gulf War Syndrome"), Chinese drywall, chlorinated solvents, plastic smell, chlorine, damp buildings, dioxin, formaldehyde, gasoline, heavy metals, herbicides, indoor air pollution, lead, lithium, manganese, mercury, metals, mold, opiates, paint, paint remover, pentachlorophenol, pesticides, phenolic resins, polychlorinated biphenyl (PCB), psychiatric drugs like anti-depressants, anti-psychotics, tranquilizers, sleep drugs, smoke removing agents, solvents, styrene, synthetic carpets, TDI toluene, welding fumes, wood preservatives, xylene, etc.

Conditions associated with neurotoxins are: *Anxiety disorder, attention deficit disorder, chemical sensitivity syndrome, chronic fatigue, dementia, developmental delay, environmental illness, hyperactivity, insomnia, memory dysfunction, mental retardation, fragrance allergy, sick building syndrome, myoclonus,* *disorders, multiple sclerosis, paralysis, panic disorder, Parkinson's disease, personality disorders, depression, psychosis, schizophrenia, sleep apnea, sleep disorder, tremors, etc.*

Neurotoxicity is a cause of brain disturbance. *Common symptoms can include problems with memory, concentration, reaction time, sleep, thinking, language, as well as depression, confusion, personality changes, fatigue, and numbness of the hands and feet.*

Almost every inhaled neurotoxin is also a lung irritant and is responsible for much asthma and other lung problems.

Neurotoxic dryer sheets are the number one cause of unregulated air pollution and really toxic. Why wash your clothes and then cover them in toxins?

Problems with the nervous system and brain are rampant. Learn to care for your brain by eating healthy fats, detoxing, relaxing, taking downtime, sleeping, and meditating. Great advances have been made in neuroscience and neuro-connectivity. It is possible to care for and make your brain better functioning at any age.

Eve Hennessa

6 CLEANING CHEMICALS

Everyone is starting to hear about how cleaning supplies are toxic. Just about every commercial cleaning product, except Bon Ami, is toxic to your health and to the environment. Keeping your home clean with baking soda, vinegar, non-toxic dish soap, and a good scrubber works as well as all of the chemicals you can buy at the store. You save money, your health, and the environment.

I will never forget when I figured out it was EASY to clean my oven with steel wool and warm water. There was never any reason to spray highly toxic solvent in there to clean it. That solvent gets into the air and later into your food.

I had stains on my tub and was amazed how my cleaning helper scrubbed them off with the rough end of a large dish sponge. I had poured bleach and every chemical in there to get rid of the stains. I have used the dish scrubber ever since and my tub is always white.

Bon Ami is a wonderful cleaner containing coconut oil, corn oil, feldspar and limestone. a natural mineral. The pesticides from corn oil are an issue for nature, but relatively non-toxic.

Tea Tree oil is a great smelling anti bacterial, anti-viral. anti fungal, anti mold. Add a few drops to soapy water. Vinegar kills all germs.

You can buy non-toxic cleaning materials. However, most products that are sold as green, organic, and healthy are not. As soon as a company becomes profitable and popular, it is bought out by a big corporation. Soon the formula changes to contain cheap chemicals.

"Green washing" is when toxic products are advertised as "natural", but are actually toxic. Mrs. Meyers and Method are now toxic. They were great products years ago when they started, but were sold to big corporations and changed. Just because Whole Foods sells it, doesn't mean it's not toxic or non-GMO! It is going to be lot better than other products, but it's best to know what's what whenever possible.

The label isn't information enough to know if something is non-toxic. These products are not regulated and the formulas are not required to be disclosed on the label. That is unless it's certified organic.

To make your home smell delicious, keep it clean and simmer some cinnamon (which also inhibits mold). Use other herbs or ORGANIC essential oils that will make your place smell great. Grow flowering plants and herbs, or find scents you are sure are non-toxic.

Sadly, lots of the natural aromatherapy machines are heating up plastics and aluminum which is toxic. Also, most of these 'essential oils' or 'natural scents' are not natural. Use certified organic if you can. Young Living Oils are toxic. Detoxing requires you to start to really learn about products. Many products which have the most hype and claims of health, often are well marketed products with cheap toxic materials.

I use non-toxic dish washing soap and can clean most things with that and a sponge with a scouring side. Once you learn how to clean this way, you realize that all of those millions of extra strength products really are not more useful than a tiny bit of scrubbing. And it's a bit of needed exercise!

Even storing all of those cleaning products adds to the toxins in your home's air. They are getting into the air. Just smell that cabinet! **If you can smell it, it's getting into your blood stream.**

When I had extreme chemical sensitivity, I would toxicity reactions being near to someones cleaning product storage closet. There is no reason to have that in your home contributing to indoor air pollution.

There is no benefit to using chemicals. The chemicals that don't make it into our blood stream go down the drain and into the water supply. Then they come back in our drinking or shower water . I just read an article that salmon from the Oregon sea were contaminated with pharmaceuticals from treated wastewater. They had anti-depressants, birth control pills, cholesterol medication etc.

I have not used a toxic chemical to clean something for years!

7 HOME AND HOUSEHOLD MATERIALS

Sick Building Syndrome and indoor air pollution are far worse than outdoor air pollution. In order for me to recover from chemical sensitivity, I had to get rid of the toxins in my apartment as much as possible. The air that I have now in my place is noticeably fresher and cleaner as compared to any other place that I visit. Your home can be a non-toxic oasis where your body can relax and recover from whatever you encounter out there in the world.

Who knew that furniture, paint, and carpet are full of toxins? They usually off-gas in three years, making them much less toxic, but some toxins do linger longer than others.

OFF-GASSING or OUT-GASSING refers to the release of airborne particulates or chemicals into the air. A really good example is if you go to Walmart or other large stores full of new stuff and smell that smell of new things. Those are plastics and all kinds of other toxins off-gassing. It's one reason people feel so unhappy in there. It's the neurotoxins!

So when you smell new furniture, new car, plastics, or new paint, that is off-gassing. Over time the toxicity of most chemicals lessens.

Here are some important things to consider in detoxing your home:

Eve Hennessa

- Dust is full of toxins like jet fuel, pesticides, mold, mites, and allergens. Keeping your home as dust-free as possible is a big help. I got rid of excess books and other items that collect dust to help reduce toxins from dust in my home.

- Shoes track in everything from lead, pesticides, jet fuel, and fecal matter into your home. Leaving shoes by the door is very helpful.

- New Carpet can be extremely toxic with some deadly chemicals. All carpets collect dust and toxins. If you have carpets, steam clean them with vinegar and keep them clean and aired.

- Particle board in furniture is toxic. IKEA is quite a toxic place! (You can seal it with a non-toxic sealant made by Safecoat).

- House Paints with VOCs and chemical fungicides are a source of poor air quality.

 Many paints that are "NO VOC" still have fungicides and other toxins. Spend the extra money to buy non-toxic paint.

- Bedding and furniture have toxic flame retardant and other toxic chemicals. Cover your mattress with old cotton blankets and top with organic sheets for better sleep conditions.

- Vinyl and other flooring is toxic.

- Plastics are off-gassing toxins in shower curtains, window shades, containers, toys, and other plastic items.

- Heating and air-conditioning ducts that are dusty, or have heated up plastics and metals, are toxic.

- Mold and mildew

Make sure you open your windows a few times every day to exchange the air. Air filters and certain air cleaning house plants have been proven to eliminate toxins from the air. Make sure your place gets sunshine and flow of oxygen. These are the things they did in the old days to make sure molds and dust mites did not take over. Sadly, modern advertising has convinced people that spraying a disinfectant is the answer. You are just spraying toxins into your home. Excessive disinfectants just create 'super-bugs'.

Those commercials and ads are asking you to poison yourself and your home.

Sunshine and oxygen are proven to inhibit mold and keep your home fresher and cleaner. UV plant lights or other UV light or even black lights can help prevent mold and mites.

8 CLOTHING

Clothing is one of the ways many toxins enter a person's blood stream. There are the chemicals in the clothes and the chemicals we wash them in. They are in very close contact with our skin and lungs.

Have you ever been into a clothing store and noticed the smell? Well that is the smell of toxic chemicals. These chemicals can get into your blood stream through the skin and through inhalation. The skin is permeable. This is why more medicines are being applied via skin patches.

Most clothing made in China is treated with pesticides and formaldehyde for shipping. So wash your new clothes at least twice before wearing. Wash until the new smell is gone. The clothing itself has plenty of toxic chemicals and pesticides. There is also Teflon and flame retardant in sporting clothes. These chemicals are particularly difficult to detox from the body. So it's best not to let them get in!

I use organic cotton sheets and also lounge around in organic clothing. When we sleep at night our body is repairing. It is a very healthy detox to sleep in a non-toxic environment.

More and more nice clothes are being made with natural fibers. Modern cotton is GMO, and GMO crops are famous for using very heavy toxic pesticides. Avoid stain-resistant and water-resistant clothing.

Detox With Ease-

Just to reiterate, washing your clothes in scented and toxic detergents and fabric sheets makes them quite toxic. Changing to non-toxic laundry detergent is one of the very best ways to detox your body! Just a cup of plain baking soda will clean clothes fine! If you want them to bubble and smell, there are non-toxic options available. I don't use fabric softener, but there are non-toxic versions.

So many people now are having 'allergies' to laundry detergents. These rashes are really your skin eliminating toxins. The skin is a detox organ and the epidemic of skin rashes and conditions is usually related to toxic chemicals.

Traditional dry cleaning is very toxic. Dry cleaners and gas stations are toxic areas. I just hand wash my *Dry Clean Only* clothes and hope for the best. I have heard that organic dry cleaning is toxic too, but have not investigated it. So far I have done pretty well washing my dry clean clothes. I have heard some people take clothes in just to be pressed.

Eve Hennessa

9 PERSONAL CARE PRODUCTS AND MAKE-UP

The average adult uses nine personal care products each day, containing 146 different chemicals. Toxic chemicals can enter the blood stream via the skin and nose. Everything that you put on your skin and hair can increase your toxic load.

These ingredients are not regulated because you don't ingest them. Since most people are not aware of how the accumulation of toxic chemicals affects the body, most industry has no concern for this whatsoever.

The Environmental Working Group regularly tests personal care products and make-up and rates them on toxicity. Please investigate your favorite products yearly.

Large corporations buy almost every natural and non-toxic product as soon as they become profitable. The corporation changes the formula and adds cheap toxic ingredients from overseas.

Women have a much higher rate of many toxic illnesses and I suspect it's the beauty products and beauty treatments like implants, lead in lip color, Botox, smelly and toxic hair products, perfumes, keratin, hair dye, nail color, etc.

The good news is that ingredients like coconut oil, minerals, herbs, and essential oils are actually nutrition for your body. More great products are coming onto the market daily.

Protect your beauty and spend that extra money on quality ingredients whenever possible!

10 DENTISTRY

Mercury is one of the most toxic substances on Earth. Never let a dentist convince you otherwise. Mercury amalgams have caused toxicity in many people.

Find a "bio dentist" who can remove these in a highly controlled way. It is important to research who removes your amalgams because removing them can cause the release of mercury into your body. It will then lodge somewhere else in your body and some people become quite ill.

There are many toxins like aluminum, BPA, and others in composite filling materials. Research this before using them. It is best to use a "bio-dentist" who uses non-toxic materials. Some are less toxic than others. There are books on how to heal cavities, but this is best done before they get too big.

Some people say that a root canal can contribute to poor health. The premise being that you have a dead tooth in your mouth which can attract bacteria. I heard that implants are not as bad.

It is possible to get well and be healthy even if you can't afford to remove your mercury. It is good to get it taken care of, but great health can be had even with mercury in the mouth. I see a lot of people on the internet really worried about the mercury. It is a concern, and can contribute to a toxic state and illness. However, there are hundred-year-olds with mercury amalgams. Oil pulling is great for detoxing the mouth and sinuses. I made a how-to video about that.

11 ENDOCRINE DISRUPTORS AND YOUR HORMONES

Endocrine disruptors are also known as hormone disruptors and estrogen mimickers. Your hormones are the messengers in the body. They keep all of the systems in your body functioning smoothly. This includes your heart, your weight, your sexual function, and your mood. Hormone imbalance, excess, or deficiency is usually a factor in almost any illness.

In order to stay healthy and happy, it is best to avoid and to detox common endocrine disruptors.

Hormone imbalance caused by endocrine disruptors is epidemic. It is an underlying cause in obesity, breast cancer, prostate cancer, and reproductive system cancers. It is also responsible for "man boobs", some erectile dysfunction, depression, anxiety, infertility, and chronic conditions. The epidemic of thyroid problems and Vitamin D deficiency are hormonal issues.

BPA is the most widely studied endocrine disruptor and has been shown to cause cancer and many other hormonal issues.

BPA is found in plastics, grocery receipts, paper money, and certain other papers. Phthalates are also endocrine disruptors. ALL plastics have endocrine disruptors. So "BPA FREE" and "PHTHALATE FREE" are better than nothing, however, all plastics made from petroleum or corn that has been heavily sprayed with pesticides are toxic and should be avoided whenever possible.

Other common Endocrine Disruptors:

- Soy is a natural estrogen boost and should not be over used by certain people.

- Drinking water has many hormone residues from pharmaceutical drugs that make their way into the water supply.

- Parabens found in lotions, shampoos, and personal care products are endocrine disruptors.

- Birth control pills and synthetic hormone replacement

- Pesticides and herbicides

- Fire retardants found in carpet, furniture, sports gear, and clothing

- Mercury, lead, dioxin, atrazine, perchlorate, arsenic, PFCs, organophosphate

- Pesticides and glycol ethers

- Artificial air fresheners, dryer sheets, fabric softeners, and other synthetic fragrances

- Food and beverages in plastic packaging (non BPA)

- All conventional products made from animals are given hormones so that they grow fast. They should be avoided. That is all 'conventional' meat and dairy. European cheeses, butter, and other products are still healthy, but check frequently because the laws change often. Lamb is usually hormone free.

12 ELECTROMAGNETIC FREQUENCIES AND RADIO WAVES

This new ubiquitous form of toxicity and source of inflammation in the body is something we should all consider and minimize in order to stay optimally healthy.

After recovering from debilitating chemical sensitivity, I was having other strange symptoms and discovered it was the electromagnetic frequencies (EMFs). EMFs cause inflammation and lots of other unwanted physical reactions, and have a strong effect on the nervous system. They are known to cause cancer.

Symptoms: Listed from the World Health Organization

- Redness

- Tingling

- Burning sensations

- Bothered by sounds

- Fatigue

- Tiredness

- Concentration difficulties

- Dizziness, nausea

- Heart palpitation

- Digestive disturbances

- Anxiety and nervous system disorders

I had some of those, plus: pressure in my head, teeth grinding, stressed out body and mind, pain in leg when using an iPad, and pain in my hand when using the computer. It was not carpel tunnel, but from the electricity. I was stressed out when in the presence of high EMFs.

These were greatly reduced by turning off my Wi-Fi and taking other measures to reduce EMFs, such as Earthing and Grounding. A few things that you can change right now are:

- Turn off Wi-Fi and data on phone when not in use.

- Keep phone away from the body.

- Unplug electronics that are not in use.

- Minimize contact with ferrous metals (like bra under-wire, filing cabinets and things made from iron). You can make a small cut pull the wire out of your bra. I do think it may contribute to breast cancer.

- Buy a grounding pad. I have made a video on this and sell it in my online shop.

- Shield or don't use mattresses with metal box springs

- Use a salt lamp to emit negative ions that counteract the EMFs.

- Use lots of black tourmaline or rocks with quartz in them to absorb or shield EMFs coming from your computer.

- Buy grounded shoes, leather soled shoes, or make your shoes into grounded shoes. I have a video on that on my Youtube channel.

There are many shielding materials available now. I have many in my website store.

Showering and water instantly grounds you. It is one reason why it's so refreshing.

****"Earthing"** or being in actual physical contact with the Earth is great healing for EMF exposure and many other illness. I have a short video about it and there is an excellent documentary called "Grounded". Touching the ground, a rock, or tree connects you to the Earth's electromagnetic current. Swimming does too. This is known to help heal any chronic illness. I credit spending many days per week in the forest as a main help in healing my chronic illness.

This "Earthing" and being in nature has been proven scientifically to improve health and well-being.

We are all in the presence of EMF levels that have never been experienced before by humans. It does cause inflammation, cancer, and other illnesses. In order to adapt to this new situation, I do feel it is wise to stay grounded and visit nature when possible.

13 BACTERIA, YEASTS, CANDIDA, AND PARASITES

Detoxing includes minimizing harmful yeasts, bacteria, and parasites that may be living in your digestive system and body. These 'bad' bacteria produce toxins that are absorbed into the blood stream, and can also damage the lining of the digestive system. It is important to limit them so that the digestive system can heal and lighten the workload of the liver.

Anybody that is ill or out of balance will also have these elements out of balance. The gut is where the immune system resides and where most neurotransmitters are found. The gut is called the second brain and is closely related to mood.

Probiotics in supplement and food form (keifer, sauerkraut, kombucha, etc.) help immensely to balance the gut flora. These gut flora keep the balance between the 'good' and 'bad' bacteria. Oil of oregano and many other herbs help to minimize yeasts and parasites. Ginger, garlic, hot peppers, peppermint, and turmeric are anti-bacterial and anti-parasite and excellent to consider adding to your diet.

There are standard anti-parasite herb tinctures available made from black walnut, wormwood, and cloves. Take this for three weeks as directed on the bottle. This can be done every six months or year to kill parasites.

This is especially good after international travel. Fresh coconut water, from the actual coconut, is great for eliminating the bad intestinal visitors too. Coconut oil is also great!

These bacteria, yeasts, and creatures love sugars, so it is important to reduce the amount of sugar you intake. Some people go as far as eliminating fruits and grains. I have never even attempted that, but have reduced both over time. Coffee and other enemas and colon cleansing also helps to eliminate many of these offenders.

Eating healthy, clean food and minimizing toxic stress will help maintain balance. Activating the parasympathetic nervous system as in meditation will help heal the gut.

Balancing your pH is also very helpful for creating an environment that they do not thrive in. Eliminating toxins will also help.

Note on weight loss: Often time your cravings are just these critters who want sugar, carbs, or other items that they like. Reducing their number and learning how to pacify them will help with a lot with ease-oriented weight loss. It's not really you who wants the sweets! It's the critters.

14 STRESS, EMOTIONS, AND THE ENERGY FIELD

Stress releases 'natural' toxic chemicals into the body. When the 'stress response' or 'fight or flight' alarm goes off in the brain, many reactions take place in the body.

As adrenaline and cortisol flood the body, breathing speeds up. Blood flow to the digestive tract and other non-essential body functions is slowed down so that you can use all of the energy in your organs, glands, and senses in order to react to the immediate danger.

Cortisol and adrenaline are toxins in the body. A chronic state of stress compromises the immune system, the nervous system, and every system in the body. Chronic or prolonged stress allows toxins to clog up the organs, which limits your capacity to efficiently eliminate toxins.

Remember, your liver, kidneys, skin, and lungs are major detox organs. Reducing stress and doing mind/body exercises by activating the parasympathetic nervous system (relaxation response) will do much to help you detox chemicals and stress from your life and body. Having your body/mind/nervous system in balance is perhaps the best way to detox. When you are in balance, the body can efficiently do its work to process toxins encountered during the day.

Once something goes wrong in the system it can be a snowball effect. Stress strongly affects the gut, where the immune system and most of the serotonin (happy mood hormones) are, and where we extract nutrition from our food. That's why so many experts say that the healing any illness *starts in the gut.*

Yoga and meditation use deep breathing, which relaxes the body, and also activates the parasympathetic nervous system. I believe that the yoga craze is really an evolutionary adaptation to the stressful life we have these days. Find the right type of yoga and teacher for you. There is a lot out there and should be something you like. I have available a daily yoga/visualization/meditation program on Skype.

Martial arts and energy exercises like tai chi are great. Any exercise that you enjoy is the right exercise! For some, boxing is appropriate. Dance has helped me tremendously.

Other activities that reduce stress and promote healthy natural chemicals are: massage, enjoying nature, singing, dancing, sex, laughing, eating, resting, playing with pets, sleeping, and friends. Any pleasurable thing that you enjoy is going to help you detox and lessen toxic stress. It seems too easy, but is probably the most healing thing you can do.

Consider letting go of people and situations that cause undue stress. I haven't watched the "news" for years. I find it distressing. Enjoying your life is not selfish but is health promoting and creates a healthy environment for everyone. Being at your best gives you the energy to help others. Being selfish with your self-care is the most unselfish thing you can do. Take time for your body and to enjoy life as much as you can.

Stress takes a lot of energy. De-stress to get that energy back. Your body needs that energy to process toxins and to be healthy and happy.

Emotional Toxins

Most cultures have long understood that the emotions are directly related to health. It has only been in the last 100 years that western science had diminished their importance in illness. There is a reason some relationships are called "toxic". They are emitting a poison that is seeping in to contaminate other areas of your life. Your physical health is no less affected. Toxic emotions are some of the most dangerous poisons.

Back when I was so ill, I started noticing that a certain 'friend' would be negative toward me and my stomach would always start to hurt. I started ending the conversation at that point and soon, he stopped saying those things. I learned that I am very sensitive to negativity of all kinds and chose to honor that.

It's a great thing to look at your relationships and change the terms and conditions more to your liking. I have more self-sufficient, functional, low-drama, and loving close friends now; this has greatly reduced my toxic load.

Mental Toxins

Thoughts and words increase acidity in the body, which creates a state of toxicity. I think it wise to not watch, read, or engage in unnecessary conversations about violence, darkness, and depressing themes. Consider whether you really need fear-inducing news and media in your life. You don't have to have a news blackout like I do, but to listen to lots of sensationalized news is incredibly toxic.

Doomsday scenarios, unfriendly gossip and other useless forms of negativity are proven to have negative effects on your health and just don't make for a fun daily life.

The body works better and can processes toxins when we have the happiness chemicals working in our favor.

It is a great detox to take a look into your mind and see what your most toxic and bad feeling thoughts are. It's often not easy to get rid of them, but there are many techniques now. There is energy clearing, neural retraining meditations, therapy, EMDR, NLP, and other help to get those minimized. YouTube has a video for everything and there are lots of great meditations on there.

Energetic Body and Spiritual Detoxification

Beside the physical body, the mind, and the emotional body, there is the energetic body, which could include the spirit, the chakras, and other energetic forces. The mind, the spirit, and the body work together simultaneously. When one heals, the others heal along with it.

It is worthwhile to learn about the energy "field" that we have around our bodies. Healing my energy field and emotions were a very important element in healing the chronic illness that I had. I also had to get rid of the synthetic toxins, but that wasn't enough for my healing. I do energy exercises every day. It has lots of great side-benefits.

Let me share a very helpful energy protection mediation I do every day. It may sound simplistic, but it changed my life.

I imagine myself sitting in an obsidian globe surrounded by a rainbow. Anything that comes in is filtered by the rainbow and the obsidian. I am now able to tolerate all kinds of electromagnetic, psychic, and emotional energy from people and places that I used to be bothered by.

I do a lot of "energy clearing" and have made a video on that. This is a big subject, but if you are reading this book, you are already on a journey toward health and this may be very helpful. Too many people are finding health and healing in this to call it 'woo-woo' any longer. It is science. Quantum physics and 'pseudo-science' is over one hundred years old, can be easily explained, and is being proven scientifically. Science that does not include the energetic is out-dated.

I have an excellent mind/body program that I facilitate on group video chat (like Skype). Find any kind of daily practice that works to keep you centered, grounded and in your body. There are many people that can help you with this.

Note on Fluoride and the Pineal Gland: The pineal gland is where the 'third eye' is located. It is widely believed that fluoride in drinking water calcifies the pineal gland and causes it to lose its function. This inner vision and intuitive function can be very handy. Many of us are able to see and heal energies using that third eye.

15 DETOX THERAPIES AND CONSIDERATIONS

Heat Therapy-Sauna

High heat from a traditional sauna, infrared sauna, sweat lodge, or hot bath is one of the most effective ways to release toxins from the body and particularly the fat cells. Fat stores toxins in order to protect your organs from storing them. This is one of the main reasons for the obesity epidemic.

Heating up the body reduces viruses, yeasts, tumors, and other toxins. It stimulates the lymphatic detox system and is excellent for the circulation. It also relaxes the body and stimulates the parasympathetic nervous system, which is very healing for the body. It is incredible! In a nutshell, sauna heat therapy cleans and detoxes the body in a way that nothing else can. It purifies the nervous and immune systems, and sweats toxins out. Almost every ancient culture had this detoxifying, purifying, and healthy practice.

Make sure your sauna in non-toxic. I advertise one that I have found to be the most safe, non-toxic and low EMF. There are lots of spas and people selling infrared sauna treatment. This is great, but the traditional heated rocks sauna is wonderful too. Most gyms have one. Just make sure they are not spraying chemical fungicides in there and that there are not plastics or toxic materials inside of the sauna.

My gym started spraying a very toxic chemical in our sauna. That is counterproductive and will make you more toxic! Luckily, they saw reason and changed the product.

Sauna is known to shrink cancer tumors. I have known people who used it for that effectively.

Colon Cleanse and Coffee Enema

One of the most effective and quickest ways to detox the body is by cleaning the intestinal tract. This is beneficial as it can remove a large amount of toxic material from the bowel quickly, reducing the risk of side effects during the detoxification process.

Coffee enema cleans the liver and also stimulates the production of glutathione, the body's own "detox molecule". Glutathione is a wonderful aid to detox, also being used as an anti-aging therapy these days. The coffee enema is the basis of the Gerson Therapy which many have used to cure cancer. Chemicals called carcinogens cause cancer and detoxing cures cancer. It is so simple. Why not detox while relatively healthy? That's my cancer motto. Do the cancer cures before becoming ill. If you are ill, detox is a great part of becoming well.

There are warnings and negative stories about coffee enemas on the internet. I thoroughly investigated them and hundreds of other positive stories before embarking on my own coffee enema protocol. People have been safely doing enemas for thousands of years. There is only one or two negative stories that circulate everywhere, and thousands of positive lifesaving results. It may be scary at first, but you get used to the enema soon enough.

When I was ill, I did almost daily coffee enemas. I believe it was the most powerful part of my detox healing regime. I would not have healed without it. Even then, it took many months for my health to turn around. I got instant relief with coffee enema after any toxic exposure reaction I had in those days.

Coffee enemas changed the health of my system over time by releasing toxins, yeasts, candida, and parasites, cleaning the liver, and stimulating glutathione (detox molecule) production. Nobody wants to talk about enemas, but they are curing cancer and doing other miraculous things.

Watch my two funny YouTube videos on the enema and coffee enema. I sometimes offer online classes or consulting on this.

There are some therapies like psyllium husk and bentonite clay drinks that clean the intestines. I prefer buying the ingredients organic and separately, rather than in a box. This will save money and increase the quality of the product, even though many products claim they have superior formulations. A little education will save time, money, and health in the long run. Some fancy packaged, natural looking health supplement may be an under-regulated Chinese import. I think it is best to stick with the known.

Different people use plants and minerals in various formulations for detox. It's not an exact science. I like to read the ingredient information of detox and colon cleansing products in order to educate myself about what is used for this purpose. There are various herbs and plants that are helpful.

If you are doing a concentrated detox by using supplements or juicing, it is helpful to do coffee enemas or other colon cleansing so that the toxins that are released will leave the body through the intestinal tract as quickly as possible. This is essential if you have any kind of illness. It is very possible to release toxins from the tissues and then can relocate and lodge in a different area of the body.

It is possible to become ill while detoxing too quickly. Colon cleansing is very helpful for this and is essential if you have a toxicity related illness or are doing an intensive detox.

Colonics are usually done professionally, however you can buy the equipment and do it yourself. Coffee enema is usually done in the home and is very simple and safe. Check with a doctor if you have diverticulitis, or other inflammatory bowel conditions. Colon cleansing may need to be supervised in these instances.

Detox Supplements

There are quite a number of supplements that aid in the detoxification process.

Detox With Ease-

One great combination is called the **"Detox Cocktail" Its:**

Alpha Lipoic Acid 300mg

Glutathione 300 mg

Vitamin C 1000

Twice a day.

You don't need to mix them together and can take other amounts. This is just a recommendation. Molybdenum is a great supplement that can help neutralize certain toxins immediately. MSM is a good one. NAC, D3, magnesium, selenium, calcium, and B vitamins are very helpful.

Correcting what vitamins, minerals, enzymes, etc. that you may have a deficiency in can help your body become more efficient in processing toxins. A body operating at optimum health will detox more efficiently.

Bentonite clay, activated charcoal, and chlorella are great for mopping toxins from the body.

I took many supplements for a while when my body was ill. Now that I am healthy, I use super-foods instead. I take a few supplements now and then as I feel I might need them.

Supplements often contain GMOs and other toxins and can possibly alter the body chemistry. I think supplements are a great help for a time and good to use intermittently. I am a believer in natural balance.

My acupuncturist taught me about this. The body is an incredible healer, and sometimes gently coaxing it to perform at a higher level of health will bring about more permanent results. As an American, I am always thinking *more is better*, but that is not usually true.

I think it is important to add as many super-foods to the diet as possible. Usually the fresher a food is the more super it is. Vitamins and minerals are just the tip of the iceberg in nutrition. Science discovers more chemical and electromagnetic properties in foods every day. Don't let anyone tell you a white potato is just starch. It is full of nutrition. All foods have properties yet to be explored. There are many wonderful properties in every fruit, vegetable, and edible root.

Glutathione suppository, IV or nebulized, is a great immediate detox. High doses of vitamin C and vitamin C drip are a strong detox, and also used for healing cancer.

In my Amazon store, detoxthebodymcs.com/shop, *you can get available supplement formulations. They are liquid, made from the best organic plant-based ingredients. They are calibrated to have the most beneficial electromagnetic properties. I know the scientist personally. They have a great brain, anti-aging, gene activator and more. I have partnered with a company from Arizona that uses Ayurveda and the latest top science.*

Detox With Ease-

Acid/Alkaline Balance

The balance of acid and alkaline in your body needs to be maintained for optimal health and detoxification. Most of us have a slightly acidic system, which can impair detoxification capacity.

Having your body at a 7 or 7.5 pH level will help enhance toxin excretion. This pH level oxygenates your body which helps in all healing. Lemon or lime water is a great alkalizer, as is sodium bicarbonate (baking soda). Excess sugars and carbs can create an acidic state.

There are books and lists of foods that can help keep your pH balance optimal. I don't think it is necessary to follow the diet in the book exactly. But it's very helpful to gain insight in how to improve your pH balance. I think it's important to be aware of your pH level. The process of balancing the body's pH has healed many toxic conditions as well as other illnesses (like cancer). You can buy pH test strips to test your urine to help you know what level you are at.

I do feel that any time you don't feel well, you are likely acidic and usually sodium bicarbonate (baking soda) or lemon water can help you feel better fast. Excess negative thoughts or emotions can cause an acidic state.

I have used the "cancer cure" sodium bicarbonate protocol to get rid of excess fungus and balance my pH. I think it helped a lot to balance my health.

Other Therapies

Detox baths, detox massages, acupuncture, and oil pulling are a few more therapies that you may want to investigate. Epsom salts are very detoxifying, and a great way for the body to absorb magnesium. Make a bath with epsom salts, organic essential oils, and a little baking soda for a great detox. Use a shower or bath filter if possible.

Oil pulling is swishing oil around between the teeth, and is a great detox. (See my video). There are liver cleanses and gall bladder cleanses. I have studied them but never felt that was for me. Perhaps a gentler version than the ones I read about would be helpful.

Minerals

We need lots of minerals in order to detox properly. Minerals help every system in the body. Modern food is lacking in minerals due to mass farming practices that deplete the soil. One great way to get minerals is to change to unprocessed sea salt. I use delicious Himalaya pink salt, which comes from ancient salt deposits in the Himalayas. Some people like other sea salts better. I prefer the ancient Himalaya salt that is found in the mountains, rather than some ocean salts that modern pollutants can contaminate. Use this to replace your 'table salt', which is chemically processed and depleted of minerals.

Bone broth soups are a great way to get minerals. Use meat from healthy farm raised animals fed non-GMO foods and not drugged with antibiotics and hormones.

Eating lots of super foods like raw chocolate, seeds, nuts, veggies, and herbs will ensure that you get lots of minerals. Many people, especially those who are ill, are not absorbing nutrients from their food. Things like epsom salt baths and other types of detox baths and oils rubbed on the skin are really helpful. Coconut oil is very healing to use on the skin and ingest. Organic essential oils are great too.

Selenium and magnesium are two important minerals that most people are deficient in. The epsom salt baths and eating cacao (chocolate) is great for magnesium. Brazil nuts are great for selenium, another essential mineral that many people are deficient in.

Probiotics

These good gut bacteria called probiotics create a number of healthy actions. These include controlling the growth of the bad bacteria, reducing inflammation, and helping you absorb nutrients effectively. Once established, they protect your digestion and remove invading organisms. If you eat a healthy diet and avoid stress and medications like antibiotics, probiotics will thrive in your digestive system and help keep you healthy.

You can take a top reputable supplement at first, but most people these days are using keifer, kombucha, and fermented foods like sauerkraut, kimchee, miso, and more to keep the gut health in good shape.

Most of the immune system is found in the gut. Serotonin (happy hormone) and a large number of neurotransmitters are found there as well. That is why healing the gut is crucial to health and well-being and why an unhealthy gut is associated with emotional, neurological, and brain function problems. GMO foods and modern wheat products are said to diminish gut health. The way I avoid GMOS is to make my own food and eat mostly organic. *Frankly, I am not comfortable being a GMO guinea pig.*

Herbs

Herbs are packed with nutrients and healing properties. There are many herbs that are effective at detoxing the body. Almost any herb in small quantities is going to have a healthy effect.

* Cilantro cleans heavy metals from the body.

* Dandelion is a great detox and immune system boost.

* Chamomile tea supports detoxification by flushing the gall bladder.

Detox With Ease-

* Peppermint soothes the digestive tract.

*Milk thistle is a potent liver detox.

* Stinging nettle, eucalyptus, and alfalfa leaf all have properties that help the body rid itself of unwanted toxins and microorganisms.

* Rosemary boosts the functioning of the liver by deactivating dangerous toxins that accumulate in your body and helping to flush them out of the liver.

Try lots of different herbs and herbal teas (skip the tea bag which contains bleaches and toxins). Your body will tell you which one it likes best at any given moment. Just use what tastes good and in the quantities you feel are 'right'.

The body feels an instinctive pull toward what it needs at any given moment. Learning to listen to your body is of great benefit.

Eve Hennessa

16 DETOX SIDE EFFECTS: HERXHEIMER EFFECT OR HEALING CRISIS

Some people experience adverse symptoms during detoxification such as nausea, changes in bowel function, or headaches. Generally these are short-term and will resolve without any intervention. However, discuss them with your practitioner if they are severe or last for more than a week.

People with severe Multiple Chemical Sensitivity, other toxicity related illness, or serious illness can have serious side effects and should always start slow while detoxing. Do a small test run on any new therapy you try. Some people's bodies are very sensitive.

I recommend coffee enemas, colonic, or other bowel cleanses while detoxing. You don't want to loosen a whole lot of toxins from one organ and have them take up location somewhere else in your body. I repeat this because of its importance. Make sure you are eliminating toxins with the colon cleanse/enema and lots of good water.

My philosophy is that pain and illness is your body telling you something is wrong. So I would ease up if you get symptoms. There are others who see it as a sign of healing and call it a "healing crisis". They think it's great and go even harder. Everyone will get symptoms when cleaning out the body. It's nothing to worry about, but don't overdo it.

Detox With Ease-

In detoxing you are changing your body chemistry and dislodging toxins. It is possible to hurt your health. Please don't get too radical in any of your practices! Don't take excessive herbs or try all of the detox practices at once. Watch how your body responds to a thing and proceed from there.

Eve Hennessa

17 THE QUICK FIX

That was a trick! There is no quick fix! The whole point of *Detox with Ease* is to go slow, steady, and get the job done right!

I had a friend that went on an extended fast while taking a detox supplement who had a psychotic breakdown. She had had that before, but not for many years. It was obvious that her whole system got thrown off by releasing too many toxins too fast into the blood stream. She is ok now.

I have also seen people on juice diets look heavier and less healthy a few shorts months after extended fasts. Just because you see two fat unhealthy guys in a documentary become slim and healthy by juicing doesn't mean that they will be long term. Long term fasting can mess up your metabolism. I did some four-day fasts for spiritual seeking. A recent Harvard study found that these short water fasts are known to reset the immune system.

However, new studies show that fasting for three days can reset the immune system. It is also said that not eating food helps your body to detox. This is all well and good if you can fast for three days. Personally, I don't believe in much fasting for most people. Unless you have the motivation, it is not very doable. I fast, but I am in a tent with no food and with a group of people doing the same thing in their own tents. When I tried on my own, I ate!

People like the idea of radically changing through fasting, but it usually doesn't work out that way. That usually results in a yo-yo or boomerang situation. I don't recommend fasting for losing weight or detoxing, but for rebooting the immune system.

Everyone wants a quick fix and most people think that extreme measures will greatly benefit them. This is not really true. Almost always, the gentle and long-term changes are the ones that actually work.

Spiritual Detox:

Various times I have done fasting in the woods alone for four days as part of a ceremony in a group setting. It is a Native American and indigenous tradition, often called a *vision quest*. It is a fast from food, phones, people, reading, writing, working, and all other distractions – and sometimes from water. It is not for most people, but a kind of passion of mine. I will go sit in the forest all day alone as a ceremony a few times a year. This has given my body and mind a lot of health and healing.

18 HAPPINESS AND WELL BEING

Long term detoxing is a matter of having your body working very efficiently so that it can process the daily encounter of new toxins.

Happiness will help with this. It is well documented that happy people are usually healthy people.

Happiness is a state you can accomplish when your mind/body/life are rid of debilitating anxiety producing toxins. Happiness is the natural state and, if achieved by me, can be achieved by anyone! This state of being will nourish your body and your life.

The latest available information suggests that we may become so ill as a result of so many inner wounds and unhappy thoughts. There are all kinds of ways to find a state of well-being. I believe that all who really want it will find the right path. It takes perseverance and courage, but is well rewarded.

When we are happy and breathing deeply the body tends toward heath. Just the addition of oxygen in the body will transform it to a more healthy state. Oxygen cleans, detoxes, and nourishes the whole body.

19 CONCLUSION

This is a short book with a life's worth of helpful information. Refer to it often and make small changes whenever you are able.

When you have gotten as many toxins out of your body and mind as you can, you will notice you have much more health, vitality, and happiness. You will have a clear mind and be able to get your dreams and goals accomplished.

This purification process is really enjoyable once you get used to it and you will feel like a new person. I promise you will feel so much better!

Your level of toxicity will be drastically reduced if you only do the following:

**Stop using dryer sheets and toxic laundry detergent

**Change your Teflon to stainless steel, glass, or cast iron

**Use non-toxic house cleaners, air fresheners, and perfumes

**Prepare your own food much more often

**Ease off of the stress

**Use better water

**Avoid factory meat and cheese

**Be aware of excess plastics

Eve Hennessa

**Buy organic sheets for sleeping

**Open your windows at least twice a day for 5 minutes to bring oxygen in and toxins out

**Spend the extra money for organic food and non-toxic items

**Avoid GMOs

**Don't buy so many new things. New things are generally toxic. Buy more expensive and better quality and less of it. All of those plastic tubs full of stuff adds to the toxicity of the indoor air. It usually takes three years to off-gas.

**Turn off your Wifi when not in use. Use your smart phone intelligently. Don't put it up to your head and keep it as far from your body as possible.

THE BEST DETOX IS LONG TERM REDUCTION IN TOXIC EXPOSURE!

We are living in times of unprecedented toxins, electromagnetic frequencies, stress, fear, and other unknowns. Detoxing, mind/body practices, and grounding in nature will enable us to adapt to this world. I believe that we must become the new super-humans in order to thrive in these times. *We can adapt to our environment and in so doing change it for the better!*

To detox the body is to help heal the Earth. Consider this:

Detox With Ease-

Every toxic chemical that is not used, does not go down the drain into the water (like when you do your laundry), the land, or the air. You are detoxing our beautiful Earth along with yourself!

The road to becoming a non-toxic super-human is also a road to healing the beautiful Earth we are privileged to live on and with.

Consider buying this for your friends and loved ones. Spread this awareness and information that you won't see anywhere else all together in such a simple format.

One little note about the internet. I love the internet. It has allowed all of this valuable information to get out. Also, it is full of misinformation and harmful products. Over time, I have found that the simplest and least costly things are the best healers. That is why you don't hear much about them. Detox and health are huge industries now. People sell their products or programs like they are the only solution. In my many years of study and experimenting, it has been the least expensive and simplest things that helped me the most – things like meditation and relaxation, clean water, breathing deeply, home cooked food, grounding to the Earth's electromagnetic field, baking soda, coffee enema, and eating fresh organic vegetables, herbs, and healthy fats.

I have vowed from the beginning to help people and only sell or advocate something that I believe to be very valuable help. Most of my information can be found for free on my website.

Additional Resources

Email questions or comments to Evespotofgold@gmail.com. I can't promise I have time to answer them all. I may address them in blog posts, videos, or my next book.

DetoxTheBodyMCS.com has much more detox info. It also has the link to my YouTube channel, Facebook, Twitter and social media and my consulting and other programs. In my consulting, I can go into more depth. I will write the long version of this book one day.

I have a daily Skype class for mind/body yoga along with different types of meditation/visualization and related practices.

Please share this book. It is my aim that all of our lives and social environments will become healthier, that many will learn to heal from chronic conditions, and that the Earth and all creatures will have a much cleaner environment.

Audio version available on Amazon and/or my website by August 2016

www.DetoxTheBodyMCS.com

Much love and healing your way!

Eve Hennessa

Detox With Ease-

Discounts for large quantities available. I hope that health institutions, hospitals, schools, and more will have this detox manual available. Also, I can eliminate the 'energy field' and other controversial topics if necessary. :)

Selected Bibliography

I scoured thousands of health websites daily for years on end.

My favorite blog is http://cancercompassalternateroute.com/ Studying healing cancer is full of great info for anyone who wants to be well.

American Lung Associationhttp://www.lung.org

Wellness Babe http://www.wellnessbabe.com/

Natural News http://www.naturalnews.com/ They have some very good health information. However, I stopped following them years ago due to their extreme negativity. This blog can draw you in and into quite a state of toxic fear. That's why it is so popular. Fear sells.

Books

Rogers, Sherry, *Detoxify or Die*, Prestige Pubs (December 2002),ISBN-10: 1887202048, 409 pages

Rogers, Sherry, *Wellness Against All Odds,* Publisher: Prestige Pubs; 42543rd edition (September 1994) , ISBN-10: 0961882158 384 pages

Rogers, Sherry, *Chemical Sensitivity,* Publisher: McGraw-Hill Education; (November 1, 1998) , ISBN-10: 0879836342, 48 pages

Joe Dispenza, *Breaking The Habit of Being Yourself: How to Lose*

Detox With Ease-

Your Mind and Create a New One, Publisher: Hay House; 4 Reprint edition (February 15, 2013), ISBN-10: 1401938094, 329 pages

Charlotte Gerson, *The Gerson Therapy: The Proven Nutritional Program for Cancer and Other Illnesses*, Publisher: Kensington (October 1, 2001), ISBN-10: 1575666286, 464 pages

Nena Baker, *The Body Toxic: How the Hazardous Chemistry of Everyday Things Threatens Our Health and Well-being*, Publisher: North Point Press; First Edition edition (August 5, 2008), ISBN-10: 0865477078, 288 pages

Theodore Brody, Alkalize or Die: Superior Health Through Proper Alkaline-Acid Balance, Holographic Health Inc; 1st edition (December 1, 1991), ISBN-10: 0961959533, 242 pages

Bruce Fife, *Coconut Cures: Preventing and Treating Common Health Problems with Coconut, Piccadilly Books, Limited (March 1, 2005), ISBN-10: 0941599604, 256 pages*

Douglas Adler MD, *The Respiratory System, The Little GI Book: An Easily Digestible Guide to Understanding Gastroenterology*, Publisher: Slack Incorporated; 1 edition (May 15, 2013), ISBN-10: 1617110728, 264 pages

Made in the USA
Charleston, SC
08 June 2016